Simplifying Nutritional Wealth Series

A series of small, easy to read books addressing common health issues women tend to have through their years. I have decided to mainly deal with WOMEN because we seem to throw hormones into the mix of everyday life. A lot of what we deal with and how we deal with obstacles comes from an emotional view. All we need to do is grab a hold of our hormones, keep them in balance and POOF…problem solved.

If we can understand the dynamics of controlling these hormones with nutrition, women will completely control the world they live in!! ENJOY!! Isra Girgrah Wynn

I0445881

ISBN: 978-1-312-27565-2

http://www.iwynn.net

iwynn is a registered trademark ® of
iwynn productions, llc. and Isra Girgrah
Wynn.

Acknowledgements:
Thank you to everyone who supports
my vision, especially my loving
husband, Marty Wynn. And thanks to
my children who keep me on my toes
24/7.

P.M.S. – Please Make Sense!

We know that PMS (premenstrual syndrome) affects your life by causing a disruption in your plans, and we also know about the stigma that's attached to it. PMS is such a regular occurrence for many women that they consider it a normal part of getting their period. About 85% to 97% of women of reproductive age get moderate to severe symptoms a week or two before their monthly cycle begins.

These symptoms include a range of physical and emotional changes. The biggest complaint is often mood-related, such as feeling extremely grouchy or unhappy, often to the point where family members know when your cycle is coming. Although more than 200 symptoms have been associated with PMS, the classic symptoms include abdominal bloating, breast tenderness, headaches, migraines, dizziness, cramps, fatigue, weight gain, nausea, vomiting, anxiety, food cravings,

irritability, depression, backaches, changes in appetite and emotional and behavioral symptoms.
These symptoms usually occur before menses begins and subside gradually at the onset of the period. Other menstrual symptoms like abdominal cramping and heavy bleeding can occur during menses.

While a variety of factors can influence a woman's symptoms during this time (including genetics, nutrition, medications, etc.), hormones largely control it, and getting hormones in proper balance can go a long way toward reducing symptoms.

Research has shown that the symptoms of PMS can be divided into five separate groups. Each group has a different type of hormonal imbalance and there is often an overlap between groups, meaning that it's likely you will suffer symptoms from more than one group.

PMS – A = Anxiety
PMS – C = Cravings

PMS – D = Depression
PMS – H = Hydration
PMS – DD = Dysphoric Disorder

These groups help indicate what may be going on internally, pointing out a specific hormone imbalance.
Rebalancing all hormones will be beneficial and have positive impact on PMS symptoms.

Understanding the cycle.
The 4 phases of menstrual cycle – follicular, ovulation, luteal, and menstruation – typically happen over a 28 day period, although this can vary from 24-35 days for some women. Your cycle is controlled by a sequence of hormones, with two most important and well known being estrogen and progesterone produced by the ovaries. Controlling the balance of all these hormones are four glands including your pituitary, thyroid, adrenals, and ovaries. The way these glands communicate with each other dictates if you

experience a smooth or bumpy ride each month.

Your pituitary, adrenals, and thyroid are hugely influenced by your external and internal emotional environment and their activity is challenged by short and long term stress. This ultimately results in your ovaries receiving confused messages each month, which reflects in imbalances between estrogen and progesterone. Your natural rhythm is disturbed and symptoms of PMS become pronounced and these two hormones remain out of sync.

Some of the reasons why hormones become imbalanced are: Stress, Exercise, Diet, Liver, and Gut.

Stress disrupts the communication network between the four controlling glands, resulting in an inappropriate release of hormones. Stress hormones block the formation of LH (Luteinizing Hormone) and FSH (Follicular Stimulating Hormone), reducing overall estrogen production, and causing progesterone levels to drop. This

interferes with the length and regularity
of your cycle.

Exercise releases endorphins, the
body's natural chemicals known to lift
our mood and since many PMS
symptoms are associated with changes
in mood it makes sense that
encouraging good endorphin production
through exercise can help to reduce the
severity of PMS. Exercise should be
featured in any program to combat
PMS, combining aerobic exercise with
strengthening activities like Yoga or
weights.

A **diet** high in refined or processed
foods and low in freshly prepared meals,
often means that the nutrients required
as raw materials for hormone
production, like vitamin B6, zinc,
magnesium, and omega 3's, are often
lacking. Topping up on fresh foods rich
in these nutrients helps to rebalance
hormone production. By cutting back on
refined foods and eating more good
quality protein (oily fish, lean meats),
nuts, seeds, and green leafy vegetables

you can help your body with hormone production.

The **liver** is one of the busiest organs of your body and is responsible for detoxification and elimination of externally produced toxins alongside the processing of all body hormones. If your lifestyle dictates high levels of external toxins like caffeine, alcohol, and food additives then your liver is put under added pressure and can often fall behind. Excess toxins are not properly removed from your body but instead are reabsorbed back into circulation disrupting hormone balance and creating cellular damage. By cleaning up your diet and lifestyle habits you give your liver a chance to catch up with itself and become more efficient at detoxifying toxins and processing hormones like estrogen and progesterone.

Constipation and the health of your intestines (**gut**) may not seem an obvious factor in PMS. However, regular bowel movements help remove toxins and processed hormones from your body. If you suffer from constipation then toxins and estrogen ready for excretion can be reabsorbed back into your body. This adds to an already likely hormone imbalance and further burdens your liver. Making regular bowel movements a priority helps to rebalance hormones and lift PMS. To overcome constipation increase fiber with oats, brown rice, fruit and vegetables and drink more water. Exercise is another excellent way of improving bowel regularity.

So which PMS group are you?

PMS – A

Do you suffer from anxiety? The typical hormone group associated with this group is that of high estrogen to low progesterone. Estrogen stimulates your nervous system by activating certain enzymes that trigger stress hormones called cortisol and adrenaline to be released. These two stress hormones increase feelings of anxiety and irritability. This coupled with lowered levels of the calming hormone progesterone means that anxiety type symptoms can become predominantly common if you suffer from this type of PMS.

Symptoms of PMS – A

- Anxiety
- Irritability
- Nervous tension
- Self-destructive behavior
- Mood swings
- Tension

To achieve a balance of all the hormones, patience is needed. While diet will help, other factors, such as reducing stress in your life, will help with hormone production. A lack of **magnesium** has been linked to many aspects of PMS, and may affect dopamine production, responsible for relaxing and soothing your mood. **Calcium** should also be taken to help regulate the balance between both minerals, and help improve mood.

*See appendix A for food choices.

PMS – C

Do you suffer from cravings? The typical hormone imbalance for this group is that of raised estrogen coupled with insulin imbalance. This results in sensations of increased appetite and strong cravings for particular foods, especially those that are high in sugar and starch. By giving in to your cravings you actually enhance the insulin imbalance, which creates a vicious cycle highlighting your symptoms. Studies have shown that during the days leading up to a woman's period your blood sugar balance and insulin sensitivity becomes less efficient for this group of PMS. By avoiding stimulants and foods that are high in refined sugars you can help your body control the blood sugar rollercoaster that may be underpinning your symptoms.

Symptoms of PMS – C
- Sugar cravings
- Starchy food cravings
- Chocolate cravings
- Palpitations

- Headaches
- Shakes
- Fatigue
- Increased appetite
- Energy highs & lows
- Cravings for stimulants

*See appendix B for food choices.

PMS – H

Do you swell up each month? Some women can gain up to 5-6lbs in the week before their period, mainly around the abdomen. Breasts also increase in size and can become tender and painful. Not only does this feel uncomfortable but it can also make you feel low and miserable. This swelling is caused by an increase in the amount of fluid surrounding your cells commonly known as water retention. This is thought to be due to higher levels of aldosterone, a hormone released by your adrenal glands, which makes your body retain salt and water. Whereas dopamine normally encourages the kidneys to remove salt and water, but as reduced levels of dopamine are common in PMS, this makes retention even worse.

Symptoms of PMS – H
- Breast tenderness
- Swollen breasts
- Water retention
- Swelling feet
- Swelling hands
- Abdominal bloating
- Weight gain

*See appendix C for food choices.

PMS – D
Do you suffer from monthly depression? Depression is the most common symptom for this group of PMS. It may be an area that some women feel uncomfortable admitting to, and it can completely alter your personality in the lead up to your period. The typical hormone imbalance of this group is one of low estrogen, high progesterone, and often high testosterone. Progesterone

depresses the activity of the nervous system, which in turn prompts an increase in the brain hormones that influence feelings of depression. Low levels of estrogen are associated with low levels of the brain hormone serotonin, which is responsible for generating feelings of relaxation and happiness.

Symptoms of PMS – D
- Depression
- Forgetfulness
- Confusion
- Crying spells
- Paranoia
- Poor coordination
- Feeling withdrawn
- Increase body hair
- Acne
- Aggression

*See appendix D for food choices.

PMS – DD
Do you suffer from severe emotional problems? Dysphoric Disorder is slightly

different from the other groups as it is classed as a completely separate condition and is far more severe than PMS. It affects a much smaller portion of women, usually only 3-5%, and involves emotional symptoms that severely affect quality of life for sufferers. The typical hormonal pattern is one of drastically low estrogen and serotonin levels, which means that PMDD is commonly treated with anti-depressants, such as Prozac, to help sufferers manage their symptoms. If you think this group is relevant to you then we would advise you to seek the advise of a general physician rather than trying to find relief on your own.

Symptoms of PMS – DD
- Suicidal thoughts
- Extreme depression
- Extreme emotional distress
- Psychological impairment
- Obsessive behavior
- Compulsive behavior
- Desire to harm self or others

The earlier you know the source of your PMS, the sooner you can effectively treat it. Unfortunately, traditional treatment is usually aimed at symptoms rather than at the root cause. The benefit of using natural treatment, such as herbs, minerals, and vitamins, is that symptoms are relieved because the body's equilibrium is reestablished. This means that symptom-relief is on going.

Please consult with your physician before dietary changes are made.

If menopause is defined by a single event (a woman's last period), **perimenopause** (menopause transition) is a bit less "pinpoint-able" as it refers instead to the time before menopause (anywhere from 2 to 10 years) during which the ovaries begin reducing hormone production. The result is fluctuating levels of the hormones estrogen and progesterone, which can set off emotional changes ranging from mild to mentally unhinged. This latter symptom in particular, which Dr. Oz recently talked about as "perimenopausal rage," is described by many women as a propensity toward unexpected, heightened anger or a vulnerability to more volatile emotional outbursts, even when the moment before you were cool as a cucumber. **Perimenopause** can start as early as 30's or up until a woman's 50's. Every woman is different. Perimenopause ends when a woman has gone twelve months without a having her period.

Symptoms of perimenopause include some or all of the following:

- Hot flashes
- Breast tenderness
- Worsening of PMS
- Decreased libido (sex drive)
- Fatigue
- Irregular periods
- Vaginal dryness; discomfort during sex
- Urine leakage when coughing or sneezing
- Urinary urgency (more frequent)
- Mood swings
- Difficulty sleeping

Here are a few dietary strategies that may help symptoms of perimenopause and keep you from feeling the need to reach for a button of your own.

Eliminate key triggers. Sugar, alcohol, and caffeine are three compounds in the diet that can exaggerate any hormonal symptoms, igniting a cocktail of emotions when stress is added. If your blood sugar is sky high after a donut, or your body's "fight or flight" stress response is over-activated from a mega-jolt of caffeine, you may be creating a perfect storm for that emotional rollercoaster. And while alcohol may seem to settle your nerves in the moment, overdoing it can have lingering effects on your edginess the next day. Eliminate these three things in your diet and you can often see a difference almost immediately.

Happy brain chemistry is dependent on getting adequate amounts of omega 3 in the diet, as it has been linked with better moods and lower rates of depression. The brain particularly loves DHA, a key omega 3 fat in the brain, which comprises 50% by weight of some brain cells. Enjoy at least two servings of fatty fish each week like salmon, sardines, tuna, mackerel, barramundi or bluefish to naturally include some of nature's richest sources of omega 3. Snack on one ounce of walnuts, which packs a day's worth of omega 3 in the form of alpha-linolenic acid, or ALA. Or drizzle two tablespoons of ground flaxseed or one tablespoon cold pressed flax oil on your morning bowl of oatmeal for an added boost. If you absolutely don't like fish, consider taking USP certified fish oil supplement. Of course, **be sure to check with your health care provider before adding any new supplements to your regimen**.

Beans and lentils are superfoods, which offer several benefits to women going through either perimenopause or menopause. The combo of high fiber and protein help to keep blood sugar stable longer after meals and snacks providing a nice buffer against those "mood swings within minutes" that many perimenopausal women describe. They also score high points for being low in calories, which helps women in their 40's and 50's maintain a healthy body weight during what is typically a time of creeping weight gain (metabolism can slow as women lose lean muscle mass if they are not involved in strength training). Legumes are also rich in B-complex vitamins, including Folate and B6, which serve as cofactors for enzymes involved with estrogen metabolism. Aim to include at least one cup per day (a half cup provides about 7 grams of protein). Enjoy a cup of lentil soup with green salad for lunch, simmer a pot of three bean chili, or savor French, green, or red lentils (they're tinier and more delicate) as your next side dish along grilled fish or chicken.

Some evidence suggests that soy might help thanks to the phytoestrogens that soybeans contain. Phytoestrogens are naturally occurring plant compounds that can mimic the body's own estrogen by binding to certain estrogen receptors, potentially helping your body ease through the loss of your own source of estrogen. Though they are about 1000 times weaker than regular estrogen, there is some evidence to suggest that including 2-3 servings of soy food daily may help reduce the severity of hot flashes, protect against bone loss and heart disease, and reduce your risk of breast cancer (a half cup of roasted soy nuts or edamame as a snack, or half cup of tofu in your stir fry all count as one serving). For that, it may be worth a try to see if you start feeling better after a month or two of adding soy to your diet. **Be sure to talk with your doctor first as adding soy may be contraindicated if you have family history of estrogen-sensitive cancers like breast cancer.**

Menopause is the permanent end of menstruation and fertility, defined as occurring 12 months after your last menstrual period. Menopause can happen in your 40's or 50's, but the average age is around 51.
Menopause is a natural biological process. Although is ends fertility, you can stay healthy, vital and sexual. Some women feel relieved because they no longer need to worry about pregnancy. The physical and emotional symptoms of menopause may disrupt your sleep, cause hot flashes, lower your energy or trigger anxiety or feelings of sadness and loss. Many of these symptoms associated with menopause are temporary. These are some ways to help reduce their effects:

Cool hot flashes. Dress in layers, have a cold glass of water. Avoid triggers including hot beverages, caffeine, spicy foods, alcohol, stress, hot weather, or warm room.

Decrease vaginal discomfort. Use over the counter, water based lubricants, choose products that don't contain glycerin which can cause burning or irritation in women who are sensitive to that chemical. Staying sexually active also helps by increasing blood flow to the vagina.

Get enough sleep. Avoid caffeine, which can make it hard to get to sleep, and avoid drinking too much alcohol, which can interrupt sleep. Exercise during the day, although not right before bedtime. If hot flashes disturb your sleep, you may need to find a way to manage them before you get adequate rest.

Practice relaxation techniques. Techniques such as deep breathing, paced breathing, guided imagery, massage and progressive muscle relaxation can help relieve menopausal symptoms. You can find a number of books, CDs and online offerings on different relaxation exercises.

Strengthen your pelvic floor. Pelvic floor muscle exercise, called Kegel exercises, can improve some forms of urinary incontinence.

Eat healthy. Eat a balanced diet that includes a variety of fruits, vegetables, and whole grains and that limits saturated fats, oils and sugars. Ask your provider if you need calcium or Vitamin D supplements to help meet daily requirements.

Don't smoke. Smoking increases your risk of heart disease, stroke, osteoporosis, cancer and a range of other health problems. It may also increase hot flashes and bring on earlier menopause.

Exercise regularly. Get regular physical activity or exercise on most days to help protect against heart disease, diabetes, osteoporosis and other conditions associated with aging.

Some complimentary and alternative treatments that have been or are being studied include:

Yoga. Some studies show that yoga, a combination of controlled breathing, posing, and meditation, and tai chi and qi gong, a series of slow movements and meditation, may be effective in decreasing the number of hot flashes in perimenopausal women. It's best to take a class to learn how to perform postures and the proper breathing techniques. **Acupuncture**. Acupuncture may have some temporary benefit in helping to reduce hot flashes.

You may have heard of or tried, other dietary supplements, such as red clover, kava, dong quai, DHEA, evening primrose oil, and wild yam (natural progesterone cream). **Consult with a professional when trying new products.**

APPENDIX A

Food tips for overcoming PMS – A

- Include as many freshly prepared foods as possible, high in vitamins and minerals. This provides the body with the basic building blocks for balanced hormone production.
- Take part in some form of relaxation as often as possible, such as having a bath, exercise, or just going for a walk. This helps reduce the levels of stress hormones produced, achieving a balance.
- Supplement with the herb Agnus Castus, which helps to increase progesterone production regaining hormone balance and reducing anxiety.

APPENDIX B

Food tips for overcoming PMS – C

- Swap all your refined 'white' foods like pasta, bread, and rice for their whole grain equivalent. Whole grain bread, pasta, rice and oats are all good sources of complex carbohydrates, which help to stabilize blood sugar balance.
- Include protein at each meal and snack like chicken, turkey, fish, beans, eggs, nuts and seeds as this helps buffer sugar balance.
- Cut back on stimulants, such as coffee, cigarettes and tea since these can also disrupt blood sugar balance.
- Start the day with a good breakfast, using both protein and complex carbohydrate. Good combinations are eggs on whole grain toast, smoothie or yogurt with granola and fresh whole fruit.

APPENDIX C

Food tips for overcoming PMS – H

- Reduce salt intake by cutting back on processed foods, salty snacks and avoid adding salt to your food. Salt makes your body hold onto water so the more in your diet, the more water you will retain.
- Increase your intake of magnesium, which helps to lower aldosterone. Up your intake of green vegetables, brown rice, walnuts and almonds, sunflower seeds, lentils and wheat germ all of which are high in magnesium.
- Avoid eating sugary foods, refined foods and bread to help lessen the feelings of bloatedness. These foods also contribute to weight gain.

APPENDIX D

Foods tips for overcoming PMS – D

- Increase foods rich in plant estrogens, which lift estrogen levels – flaxseeds, soy yogurt, miso. Reduce your alcohol intake to help reduce the depressive effects.
- To help regain estrogen and progesterone balance increase foods rich in vitamin B6 and Zinc. Include wheat germ, brown rice, eggs and whole grains for vitamin B6; fish, nuts and seeds for zinc.
- Include foods high in the good fats such as oily fish (salmon and mackerel), nuts and seeds. This helps to boost brain hormones, which lift mood. In fact, it's well worth supplementing with omega 3 fish oil.
- For pre-menstrual acne, aggression or increased body hair, supplementing the herb saw

palmetto can help address the
testosterone imbalance
associated with these symptoms.

APPENDIX E

Foods that are good for Fighting PMS

Fat is your friend. A mix of essential fatty acids significantly reduces PMS symptoms. Don't be shy of healthy fats (avocados, salmon, nuts, olive oil) and consider supplementing with fish oil.

B it up. A diet rich in B vitamins – meat, beans, spinach, fortified cereal and whole grains – can also help.

The calcium and vitamin D connection. Vitamin D seems to be good for everything these days, including PMS. A diet rich in calcium and vitamin D may lower the risk of developing PMS in the first place. Getting four servings of fortified orange juice or low-fat dairy foods such as yogurt each day, which adds up to about 1,200 milligrams of calcium and 400 International Units of vitamin D a day.

APPENDIX F

5 Ultimate Tips For Maintaining Female Hormone Balance

1. **Follow a well-balanced and nutrient dense diet** – fruits and vegetables, complex carbohydrates, good quality protein, nuts and seeds will all help rebalance and maintain your hormones.
2. **Include soluble fiber** such as oats, lentils, brown rice, fruit and vegetables. This will help keep your bowels regular and remove any toxins and hormones from building up.
3. **Take a multivitamin and essential fatty acid supplement** to ensure you stay topped up with all the necessary nutrients.
4. **Include some form of relaxation and/or exercise** into your weekly routine. Something like 3 sessions a week of aerobic

exercise and a yoga class is ideal. The important thing is setting time aside for you.

5. **Cut down on alcohol, caffeine, and smoking,** as these three factors cause your body extra stress as well as depleting the nutrients needed for hormone production and balance.

Top Perimenopausal Power Foods

Almonds (raw, unsalted)
Almonds are a great source of protein, fiber and minerals including:
Calcium and magnesium – calcium keeps bones strong and promotes bone growth. Magnesium works in concert with calcium for bone growth and is a calming mineral needed by perimenopausal women. It is also good for assisting with constipation.
Iron – this mineral is necessary for transporting the active and usable form of thyroid, T3.
Potassium – circulatory deficits happen with age and declining hormones; potassium ameliorates this by helping to support blood vessel health and reduce the risk of high blood pressure. A potassium rich diet will prevent leg cramps and other muscle spasms. This is because of the role that potassium plays with muscle contraction and nerve

impulses all over the body, including the heart.

Zinc – research indicates that zinc helps balance female hormones, helps prevent PMS, and helps prevent acne.

Almonds are also high in vitamin E and unsaturated fats, keeping arteries supple. With the decline of minor hormones, cortisol goes high and is one of the main reasons women get (and die of) heart disease; almonds play a role in preventing atherosclerosis (hardening of the arteries).

Apples
All types of apples contain Quercetin, a powerful antioxidant that prevents the oxidation of LDL cholesterol, which in turn lowers the risk of damage to your arteries. An apple's pectin is effective in lowering levels of blood cholesterol.

Avocado
This fruit may prevent breast cancer as well as prostate cancer.

Beans

Beans are loaded with complex carbohydrates, as well as calcium, iron, folic acid, B vitamins, zinc, potassium and magnesium. They contain large amounts of soluble and insoluble fiber, which helps reduce cholesterol and normalize blood sugar.

Beets

Beets contain high levels of carotenoids and flavonoids, which are known to protect artery walls as well as reduce the risk of heart disease and stroke. In addition, they contain iron and also boost bone health, due to their calcium content, thus reducing the risk of osteoporosis.

Blueberries

Berries are a great source of antioxidants that keep your brain and heart healthier. Blueberries also contain pterostilbene, which is effective in reducing bad LDL cholesterol.

Broccoli

This vegetable contains two powerful anticancer substances: sulforaphane and indole-3-carbinol. Sulforaphane destroys ingested carcinogenic compounds and kills H pylori (Helicobacter pylori), a bacteria that causes stomach ulcers and increases the risk of gastric cancers. (If you eat in restaurants and consume nonorganic chicken, it's likely at some point you will pick up H pylori). Indole-3-carbinol metabolizes estrogen, potentially protecting against estrogen dominance and breast cancer. It also has a good amount of potassium and beta-carotene.

Cabbage

High in fiber, vitamin A and minerals, cabbage stimulates the immune system, kills bacteria and viruses, inhibits growth of cancerous cells, protects against tumors, helps control estrogen levels and promotes balance, improves blood flow and boosts sex drive. It speeds up the metabolism of estrogen toward a "good" metabolite and slows the production of a bad one, reducing the risk of breast cancer, and inhibits the growth of polyps in the colon; cabbage also protects against stomach ulcers.

Eggs
Eggs are a good source of selenium, riboflavin, vitamin B12, pantothenic acid and vitamin D, and are rich in lutein and zeaxanthin (both offer protection for the eyes, which were not meant by nature to last beyond our childbearing years). Eggs are also a great source of choline, a neurotransmitter critical for brain health and a good source of natural progesterone.

Flaxseed
This power food increases the number of ovulatory cycles in perimenopausal women and increases testosterone at the time of ovulation. Regular consumption of flaxseed improves the progesterone/estrogen ratio in postovulatory women and helps with PMS. Flaxseed is also an excellent

source of essential omega-3 fatty acids. Freshly ground flaxseed releases more nutrients than whole flaxseed.

Garlic
This yummy bulb is an excellent cancer fighter, protecting against cancers of the breast, colon, skin, prostate, stomach and esophagus. Garlic stimulates the immune system by encouraging the growth of natural killer cells that directly attack cancer cells. Also, it has the ability to kill many of the antibiotic-resistant strains of MRSA (the hospital superbug).

Meat
Lean meats (organic, of course, and grass-fed whenever possible) are an excellent source of protein. Meat also provides needed iron, B12, and zinc. Bison meat is often overlooked as an example of healthier meat, because bison live on natural grass and spend very little time in feedlots or slaughterhouses. As such, they are not given drugs, chemicals or hormones. Bison meat has a greater concentration

of iron than any other meat, as well as some essential fatty acids. Of particular importance to women is its high iron content.

Nuts

Nuts and seeds provide excellent nutritional value. They are especially good sources of essential fatty acids, gamma tocopherol, vitamin E, protein and minerals. They also provide valuable fiber components; important phytonutrients in nuts and seeds include protease inhibitors, ellagic acid and other polyphenols.

Olive Oil

Regular consumption of this omega-3 rich oil helps protect against heart attacks, because of its unique polyphenol and monounsaturated fatty acid content. Polyphenols in extra virgin olive oil help keep cell membranes soft and pliable, allowing for oxygenation and hydration, the elements of life, to flow through the membranes easily and thus give energy and vitality.

Oranges
Oranges contain high quantities of hesperetin, which protects against inflammation. Eating these regularly can lower cholesterol because of the fiber/pectin. They are a good source of potassium, which reduces blood pressure, as well as folic acid, which lowers levels of homocysteine (high levels of this substance in the body are not good for the heart).

Pineapple
This is one of the top 50 foods with the highest antioxidant content. Antioxidants have been found to help protect cells from the damage of free radicals, which can break down muscles, increase aging effects and, as a result, lead to cancers and other chronic diseases.

Shellfish
These sea gifts are full of healthful vitamins and minerals. Oysters are a great source of vitamins A, B1, B2, B3,

and D, and are also high in iron, calcium, magnesium and other minerals. Many other shellfish are also excellent sources of iron and zinc – mussels, clams, scallops, shrimp, prawns, and cab. Shellfish are one of the best dietary sources of zinc, a mineral necessary for keeping your immune system healthy and promoting the healing of wounds. The highest levels of zinc can be found in oysters.

Sweet Potatoes
This power food is full of protein, fiber, artery-protecting beta-carotene, blood pressure-controlling potassium, and antioxidants.

Tea
Black, green and now white teas are hailed for their anti-oxidant properties. The polyphenols in green tea are powerful antioxidants and protect against free radical damage, which is a major cause of arterial aging. Green tea

may inhibit breast, digestive and lung cancers as well.

Tomatoes
Cooked tomatoes contain high levels of lycopene, a nutrient that reduces the risk of prostate, lung and stomach cancers. Tomatoes contain potassium, vitamin C, and lycopene; each is essential to your immune system and to keep your skin healthy.

Wild Salmon
This fish is an excellent source of omega-3 fatty acids. Eating omega-3 rich salmon regularly may help protect against heart disease, breast and other cancers, as well as provide relief to sufferers of certain autoimmune diseases, such as rheumatoid arthritis and asthma. Its omega-3 are great for mood and also protect the brain, and are essential for the membranes of every one of your 60 to 90 million or so cells in your body.

Basic Dietary Guidelines For Menopause

Get enough Calcium. Eating and drinking two to four servings of dairy products and calcium rich foods a day will help ensure that you are getting enough calcium in your daily diet. Calcium is found in dairy products, fish with bones (such as sardines and canned salmon), broccoli, and legumes. An adequate intake of calcium for women aged 51 and older is 1,200 milligrams per day.

Pump up your iron intake. Eating at least three servings of iron-rich foods a day will help ensure that you are getting enough iron in your daily diet. Iron is found in lean red meat, poultry, fish, eggs, leafy green vegetables, nuts, and enriched grain products. The recommended dietary allowance for iron in older women is 8 milligrams a day.

Get enough fiber. Help yourself to foods high in fiber such as whole grain breads, cereals, pasta, rice, fresh fruits, and vegetables. Most adult women should get about 21 grams of fiber a day.

Eat fruits and vegetables. Include at least 1-½ cups of fruit and 2 cups of vegetables each day.

Read labels. Use the package label information to help you to make the best selections for a healthy lifestyle.

Drink plenty of water. This will help you stay hydrated. It's impossible to determine how much water we all need, because this depends on many factors, such as how much you eat, the climate you live in, and how active you are. As a general rule, drinking eight glasses of water every day fulfills the daily requirement for most healthy adults.

Maintain a healthy weight. Lose weight if you are overweight by cutting down on portion sizes and reducing foods high in fat, not by skipping meals. A registered dietician or your doctor can help you determine your ideal body weight.

Reduce foods high in fat. Fat should provide 25% to 35% or less of your total daily calories. Also, limit saturated fat to less than 7% of our total daily calories. Saturated fat raises cholesterol and increases your risk for heart disease. Saturated fats are found in fatty meats, whole milk, ice cream, and cheese. Limit cholesterol intake to 300 milligrams (mg) or less per day. Also try to limit your intake of trans fats, found in vegetable oils, many baked goods, and some margarines. Trans fats also raise cholesterol and increases your risk for heart disease.

Use sugar and salt in moderation. Too much sodium in the diet is linked to high blood pressure. Also, go easy on smoked, salt-cured, and charbroiled foods – these foods contain high levels of nitrates, which have been linked to cancer.

Limit alcohol intake. Women should limit their consumption of alcohol to one or fewer drinks a day.

Please consult with your physician before making any changes to your diet and exercise.

Bibliography

http://www.webmd.com
http://www.thefooddoctor.com
http://www.pms.org.uk
http://www.doctoroz.com
http://www.abcnews.go.com
http://www.mayoclinic.com

www.ingramcontent.com/pod-product-compliance
Lightning Source LLC
Chambersburg PA
CBHW070340290526
45791CB00003B/1405